ALL  Constipation

Edited by
Dr Savitri Ramaiah

New Dawn

NEW DAWN
a division of Sterling Publishers (P) Ltd.
L-10, Green Park Extension, New Delhi-110016
Ph.: 6191784, 6191785, 6191023 Fax: 91-11-6190028
E-mail: ghai@nde.vsnl.net.in
Internet: http://www.sterlingpublishers.com

Constipation
©1999, Sterling Publishers Private Limited
ISBN 81 207 2223 X
Reprint 2001

All rights are reserved. No part of this publication may be reproduced, stored in a retrieval system or transmitted, in any form or by any means, mechanical, photocopying, recording or otherwise, without prior written permission of the publisher.

Published by Sterling Publishers Pvt. Ltd., New Delhi-110016.
Lasertypeset by Vikas Compographics, New Delhi-110029.
Printed at Prolific Incorporated, New Delhi-110020.

Information for this series, has been provided by *Health Update*, a monthly bulletin of the Society for Health Education and Learning Packages. The Update is intended to provide you with knowledge to adopt preventive measures and cooperate with the doctor during illness for better outcome of treatment.

Contributors

ALLOPATHY
Dr. Rakesh Agha
(Consultant Gastroenterology, Apollo Hospital, New Delhi)

Dr. Vijay Zutshi
(Senior Consultant, Department of Obstetrics and Gynaecology, L.N.J.P. Hospital, New Delhi)

AYURVEDA
Dr. V.N. Pandey
(Director, Central Council for Research in Ayurveda and Siddha, Delhi)

HOMOEOPATHY
Dr. Poonam Jain
(Consultant Homoeopathy, Delhi)

NATURE CURE
Dr. Sambhashiva Rao
(Chief Medical Officer, Institute of Naturopathy, Bangalore)

Preface

All You Wanted to Know About is an easy-to-read reference series put together by *Health Update* and assisted by a team of medical experts who offer the latest perspectives on body health.

Each book in the series enhances your knowledge on a particular health issue. It makes you an active participant by giving multiple perspectives to choose from — allopathy, acupuncture, ayurveda, homoeopathy, nature cure and unani.

This book is intended as a home adviser but does not substitute a doctor.

The opinions are those of the contributors, and the publisher holds no responsibility.

Contents

Preafce   4
Introduction   6
Allopathy   7
Ayurveda   83
Homoeopathy   101
Nature Cure   117
Definitions   139
References   142

Introduction

Constipation is a symptom not a disease. Generally, constipation is said to exist — when the frequency of passing stool is less then three times a week.

Constipation results when their is abnormality in diet, inadequate liquids, stress and anxiety, irregular habits, lack of exercise, bad posture and medicines.

Constipation can be treated with non-medicinal as well as medicinal measures. It can be prevented and controlled by eating a high fibre diet, drinking quantities of water, regular habits, and exercises. Correct posture is crucial for passing stool.

ALLOPATHY

ALLOPATHY

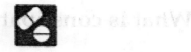

Constipation is a very common symptom. Many people suffer from it regularly and most have constipation at some point of time or the other in their life. It is important to know that often people who "feel constipated" may actually not be. Constipation can be prevented by adopting regular and suitable life-style, especially diet.

What is constipation?

It is not easy to define constipation. This is because the normal frequency of passing the stool varies considerably among people. It varies from three to eleven stools per week. Generally, constipation is said to exist when the frequency of passing stool is less than three times per week. Other criteria for defining constipation include:

- hard consistency of the stool;
- difficulty in passing the stool;

- excessive straining while passing the stool;
- heavy or full feeling in the lower abdomen; and
- feeling of incomplete passing of the stool.

How is the stool formed and passed out?

Stool is formed from the undigested food. After you swallow food, it passes through the food pipe, the stomach, and small *intestine*, in that order. The stomach acids mix with the food and result in a soft soup like consistency. Digestion of food takes place in the small intestine by chemical substances called *enzymes*. The muscles of the intestines contract and relax in rhythmic fashion

Fig 1. The Digestive System

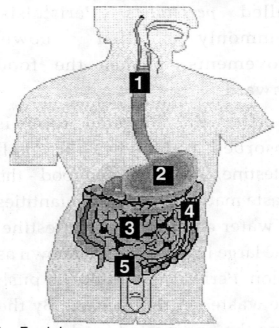

1. Food pipe
2. Stomach
3. Small Intestine
4. Large Intestine
5. Rectum

resulting in a wave like movement called *peristalsis*. Peristalsis, commonly called bowel movements, pushes the food forward.

After the digested food is absorbed by blood in the small intestine, the undigested food - the waste matter - and large quantities of water enter the large intestine. The large intestine is also known as colon. Peristalsis continue to push the waste matter forward. By the time the undigested food reaches the end of the large intestine, most of the water is absorbed and stool is formed. The last ten centimetres of the large intestine is a chamber called *rectum*. The rectum ends in an opening called *anus*. The anus is guarded by two bands of muscles which keep it in closed position. These bands are the *inner* and *outer anal sphincters*. Sphincters are circular muscles which bind an opening tightly and keep it closed or contracted.

The stool is passed from the rectum by coordinated activity of nerves and muscles of the anus and rectum. When rectum distends with the stool, the inner sphincter relaxes and the outer sphincter contracts. The outer sphincter is under voluntary control - which means that the choice to pass stool or not depends on you. This is the time when you get the urge to pass the stool. The outer sphincter responds or opens up in response to:

- voluntary effort of straining,
- manual stretching of the area around the anus, and
- distention of the rectum. Stretching of the anus and rectum also increases peristalsis in the large intestine. Increased

peristalsis pushes the stool located higher in the large intestine into the rectum. Thus, the stool in the intestine and rectum is passed out. The organs of the digestive system are shown in Figure 1.

What are the causes of constipation?

Constipation results when there is abnormality in: (1) passage of waste food through the large intestine and/or (2) coordinated activity between the rectum and anus. Slow passage of food in the large intestine allows more water to be absorbed. Increased water absorption results in hard stool. Lack of coordination between anus and rectum results either in partial evacuation or a feeling of incomplete evacuation. Detailed below are the reasons for development of constipation.

- ***Diet.*** Low fibre diet is one of the commonest causes of constipation. Low fibre diets are (1) diets with less vegetables, fruits and whole grains; and (2) diets rich in fat foods such as cheese, egg and meat. Fruits, vegetables and whole grains have soluble and insoluble fibre. The soluble fibre dissolves in the intestines to form a soft texture. This soft texture of the dissolved fibres keeps the stool soft. Insoluble fibre does not change during digestion. It is excreted as it is, thus adding bulk to the stool. Increased bulk increases peristalsis.

- *Inadequate liquids*. The stool is hard and small in volume if you drink less than eight to ten glasses of fluids such as water or fruit juices per day. Hard and small stool results in poor peristalsis and excessive straining for passing it.

- *Stress and anxiety*. Emotional stress and anxiety decrease peristalsis. In addition, people with stress tend to eat low fibre diet, often at irregular timings. Eating at irregular hours does not allow adequate time for complete digestion of food. It also results in poor peristalsis.

• *Irregular habits.* Some people tend to ignore the urge to pass stool. This is either because they are too busy or are not near a toilet of their choice at the time of the urge. The urge to pass the stool stops if you ignore it often.

• *Lack of exercise.* People with sedentary life style have poor tone of the abdominal muscles and reduced peristalsis.

• *Bad posture.* Constipation can occur if there is a wide angle between the thighs and the hips while passing the stool. This is often the case when people sit straight on a western type of toilet. People who are used to Indian toilet may develop constipation if they start using the western type of toilet.

• *Pregnancy*. Pregnant women have reduced bowel movements. Common causes of constipation in pregnancy have been elaborated in further chapters.

• *Medicines*. Common medicines also reduce peristalsis and cause constipation.

- *Old age*. Old people have constipation because (1) those who do not have teeth eat soft, low-fibre diet, (2) activity of the intestine decreases, and (3) poor muscle tone of the abdomen.

- *Travelling*. Normal diet and routine activities are disturbed during travel resulting in constipation.

- *Hirschsprung's disease*. This is a *hereditary disease* in which there are no nerves in the rectum and the two sphincters of the anus. Absence of nerves results in constriction of the rectum. This constriction causes mechanical obstruction for passage of the stool. The intestine before the constricted rectum expands to accommodate the stool which is not passed out. This expansion weakens the wall of the intestine and the stool is not passed out. Hirschsprung's disease often causes constipation very early in life.

• *Chronic diseases*. People with long-term illness have constipation due to five main reasons:

• reduced physical activity;

• reduced peristalsis as a consequence of the disease;

- reduced efficiency of the rectum and anus;

- side-effects of medicines prescribed for some chronic illnesses, and

- muscle weakness of the *"diaphragm"* and the abdomen. Diaphragm is a muscle sheet which separates the abdomen and the chest. It moves up and down when you breath.

What are the causes of constipation during pregnancy?

There is decreased peristalsis during pregnancy due to:

- *Progesterone* — a hormone — which relaxes muscles of the large intestine.
- Changes in dietary habits.
- *Mechanical compression and displacement* of the large intestine by the womb.
- Relaxation of the muscles of the abdomen.

- Increased water absorption from large intestine.
- *Changes in the normal activity* and exercise pattern.
- *Tension* and anxiety.
- *Iron* tablets or tonics.

What are the causes of constipation in children?

Constipation in newborn babies and older children have different causes. Mothers often tend to believe that children cry frequently due to constipation or colic pain. This is not always true. Also, there are several misconceptions regarding the normal frequency of the stool in a newborn. Breast-fed babies pass seven stools in a day to about a few times a week. However, it is important to rule out

Hirschsprung's disease in a child who passes few stools every week. If the child is normal, simple measures such as increasing frequency of breast feeding may increase the stool frequency. Newborn's stools will also increase if the mother eats larger quantities of citrus fruits, prunes and papaya. Medicines for increasing frequency of stools and reducing colic pain should not be given to children unless the doctor prescribes them.

Constipation in older children may be due to low fibre diet, family obsession with "regular" bowel habits, emotional causes, inadequate time in the morning to go to the toilet and ignoring the urge to pass the stool due to dirty toilets in the school.

What are the common medicines that cause constipation?

Some common medicines also cause constipation. These are:

- Pain killers.
- Non-steroidal antiinflammatory medicines.
- Antacids especially those with aluminium and calcium (medicines taken for acid burn in the stomach).
- Medicines for diarrhoea.

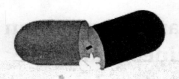

- Anaesthetic agents (medicines that cause partial or complete loss of feeling).
- Medicines for high blood pressure.
- Medicines for depression.

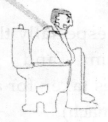

- Medicines for Parkinsonism.
- Medicines for epilepsy.
- Iron tablets and tonics.
- Diuretics (medicine that increase secretion or urine).
- Bariumsulphate used for x-ray of the stomach and intestines.
- Some medicines for treatment of constipation if taken for a long time.
- Drugs that cause addiction.

What are the common diseases that cause constipation?

Some common illnesses that cause constipation. These are:

Diseases of the nervous system:

- Hirschsprung's disease.
- Brain tumors.
- Stroke with paralysis.
- Injury to the spinal cord and nerves of the intestines.
- Multiple sclerosis: This is a progressive disease that causes

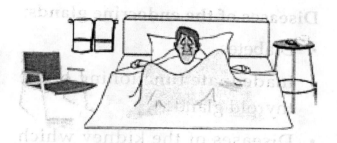

reduced or abnormal sensations in the limbs, muscle weakness, dizziness, visual disturbances, etc.

- Parkinson's disease: This disease results in involuntary movements such as tremors, muscle rigidity, slow shifting walk, difficulty in chewing, swallowing and speaking.

Diseases of the endocrine glands:
- Diabetes.
- Inadequate functioning of the thyroid gland.
- Diseases of the kidney which result in increased urea and other waste products in the blood.
- Diseases of parathyroid glands that increase calcium in the blood.

Diseases of the large intestine:
- Tumorous.
- Hernia.

- Constriction of a part of the intestine.
- Tuberculosis.
- Some cases of irritable bowel syndrome.
- Syphilis, a sexually transmitted disease.
- Surgery.

Is constipation a serious disease?

There are two types of constipation: (1) simple; and (2) severe without a known cause.

Simple constipation is usually due to inadequate and/or improper diet and life-style. People with simple constipation do not have any major illnesses. They get relief from constipation by improving their diet and/or use of substances that increase volume of the stool.

Severe constipation without any known cause usually occurs in young women. It starts in childhood or adolescence. Psychological factors play a role in this type of constipation. It may also be due to ignoring the urge to pass stool. Severe constipation without any known cause is difficult to treat. Many people with this type of constipation do not have relief even after eating high fibre diet. In fact, in some cases, high fibre diet may even worsen the symptoms. People with severe constipation without known cause have decreased peristalsis and abnormal contraction of the muscles around the anus.

Irritable bowel syndrome, a condition observed more often in young to middle aged adults can also cause constipation. Irritable bowel syndrome is a chronic disease for which no cause is known. The symptoms are:

- pain in the lower part of the abdomen;
- small, hard stool; and
- a feeling of incomplete evacuation after excessive straining.

It can also cause

- increased passing of gas from the anus,
- a bloated sensation in the abdomen,
- heartburn,
- nausea and
- back pain.

Some people with Irritable bowel syndrome have alternate constipation and diarrhoea. Anxiety increases the severity of the symptoms. In fact some people may begin to fear that they have serious diseases such as cancer. It is therefore important to reassure such people and motivate them to follow the doctor's guidelines for managing the Irritable Bowel Syndrome.

Constipation in old people can result in "false" diarrhoea. This is because dry and hard stool blocks the end of the large intestine. The liquid part of the stool above this block leaks around it and is passed as loose motions. Proper treatment of constipation relieves "false" diarrhoea.

If you **develop constipation suddenly**, consult a doctor as soon as possible. In such cases it is important to rule out obstruction in the large intestine. Causes of such obstruction are:

• *Tumours of the large intestine*. They may or may not be due to cancer;

• *Narrowing of a part of intestine* due to some diseases;

• *Foreign bodies* in the intestine;

• *Narrowing of the anus*. The anus contracts due to painful conditions such as piles or fissures; and

• *Injury*. Injury of the lower part of the backbone and nerves to the intestine result in constipation due to five main reasons:

- poor peristalsis,
- dilatation of one part of the intestines which does not allow stool to move forward,
- decreased tone of the muscles of the rectum,
- decreased sensation in the rectum so that people cannot get the urge to pass stool, and
- inadequate passing of stool due to reasons listed above.

How do I know whether my constipation is simple or serious?

More than eighty percent people have simple constipation. Your doctor is the best person to judge the causes and type of your constipation. In order to assess the cause of your constipation, or whether you have constipation or not, the doctor will ask you several questions. These include:

1. What are your normal habits for passing the stool in terms

of frequency, volume and timings?

2. What is the duration of constipation?

3. What is the consistency of the stool? Do you need to strain a lot while passing the stool? Do you have a feeling of either fullness in the abdomen or incomplete evacuation?

4. Have you ever taken medicines for constipation? If yes, for how long, and what medicines. Do these medicines relieve constipation?

5. Do you have any other complaints in the abdomen?
6. Are you normally stressed?
7. Do you take medicines regularly? If yes, how often, and what medicines?
8. Do you have any other health problems?

After taking detailed history, the doctor will examine you to find out if you have any other diseases. He/she will examine your anus for any deformity or injury around it. The doctor may also do a manual examination of the rectum to find out if there are abnormalities of the rectum such as piles, fissures, tumours, narrowing of the rectum, prolapse or hard stool lodged in the rectum. Your doctor may suggest some laboratory investigations, if necessary.

What are the complications of constipation?

The Allopathic system of medicine does not consider the stool lodged in the intestines as "poison". Common diseases caused by or aggravated by constipation are:

• *Hernia and piles*. Excessive straining for passing stool increases the pressure in the abdomen. Increased pressure can lead to hernia and worsen piles.

- *Fissures*. The passage of dry and hard stool may cause injury to the lining of the anus. This injury is called fissure and is very painful.

What are the laboratory investigations for constipation?

Laboratory investigations are necessary to rule out diseases which can cause constipation. These include:

Blood tests for

- abnormalities of the thyroid gland,
- diabetes,
- calcium levels and
- uric acid.

- *Barium enema* is a procedure in which a chemical substance called barium sulphate is pushed into the rectum and series of x-rays taken. This substance does not absorb x-rays. When the barium fills the intestine and the rectum, their shape and condition are therefore seen clearly. Barium enema is used to detect

- tumour,
- narrowing or dilatation of the intestine and
- absence of normal folds in the intestinal walls. It is a simple, painless test. There may, however,

be mild discomfort when the barium fills the intestine.

The test will not be successful if you have stool in the intestine. Your doctor will therefore prescribe a simple medicine to be taken at bed time the day before the barium enema. This medicine will result in complete evacuation of stool the next morning. You are likely to pass chalk-like stool for a few days after the barium enema.

- *Endoscopy* is a procedure for direct viewing of the rectum and the large intestine with a long tube. If the lower part of the large intestine is viewed, the procedure is called *sigmoidoscopy*. If the entire large intestine is viewed, the procedure is called *colonoscopy*. Just as in barium enema, you need to take medicines to evacuate stool completely from the intestines. Sometimes enema may be necessary the previous night and/or just before the test. Endoscopy is best done after overnight fast. The doctor may prescribe mild sedatives to reduce anxiety and help you relax during the procedure.

Before doing the endoscopy, the doctor will first examine your rectum with gloved fingers covered with a lubricating agent. He/she will then insert a long plastic endoscopic tube through the anus. As the tube is pushed into the rectum, you may feel an urge to pass stool or have a mild cramp like pain in the lower abdomen. These symptoms last only for a few minutes. There is a light at the end of endoscopic tube which enables the doctor to study inner part of the rectum and large intestine on a television screen while performing the test. Endoscopy is an ideal test for studying the condition of the intestine. The doctor will take a small part of the intestine for biopsy if there are tumours, ulcers, or other abnormalities. Endo-scopy will also indicate if constipation is due to excessive intake of some medicines for constipation.

• *Colonic transit studies* are recommended when medicines for treatment of constipation are not effective. Colonic transit studies analyse peristalsis in the large intestine. In this test, series of x-rays are taken for three to seven days after you take a capsule containing some chemical substance. This chemical substance is not absorbed in the body and is seen clearly on the x-ray. The time taken for the chemical substance to pass through the intestines is recorded through x-rays. Most people excrete about eighty percent of the chemical substance within seventy hours. Longer time indicates inadequate peristalsis. You should eat a high fibre diet during the test.

- *Anorectal function tests* are also recommended when medicines fail to relieve constipation. They are used to study

- coordinated activity of the rectum and the anus, and
- elasticity of the inner anal sphincter. This test is very useful for detecting irritable bowel syndrome, Hirschsprung's disease and those with large distended rectum. A soft paste with stool-like consistency is injected into the rectum to study *rectum and anus coordination*. X-rays of the rectum and anus are taken while you excrete the paste in a toilet seat kept inside an x-ray machine. These x-

rays detect abnormal functions of the rectum and anus. To study the *elasticity of the sphincter of the anus,* a balloon filled with air is inserted in the anus and pulled back. A special equipment is used to measure the elasticity of the sphincters as the balloon comes out.

What is the treatment for constipation?

Constipation is treated with *non-medicinal* and *medicinal measures*. It is important to remember that there is no standard treatment for constipation. Similarly, the duration of treatment varies from person to person. The doctor will decide on your treatment only after detailed history and examination. Non-medicinal measures are extremely important for prevention and control of constipation. These include:

- *Dietary fibre.* The first and the most important step in the management of constipation is increasing dietary fibre and if required, adding fibre supplements. Several studies have conclusively shown that the more the stool weight, the faster it moves through the large intestine. Fibre increases stool weight, bulk and fluidity and thus help the stool to pass out. Foods with high fibre content are wheat, corn, oats, barley, peas, dried beans, seeds, nuts, fruits and vegetables. Box 1 lists guidelines for a high fibre diet.

Box 1. Guidelines for high fibre diet

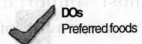
DOs
Preferred foods

Cereals: Whole wheat flour from the mill, dalia, oatmeal, brown bread, makai or bajra

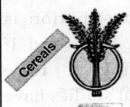

Pulses: Whole or crushed pulses or dals with skin, beans, sprouted beans, bengal gram, and kidney beans

Fruits: All fruits with peels and pips in fruits such as apple, pear. Also, watermelon, guava, goose-berries, grapes, pome-granate, plums, papaya

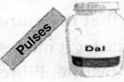

Vegetables: Raw salad, half cooked or slightly under cooked, leafy vegetables, cabbage, spinach, lettuce, tomatoes, cucumber, brinjal

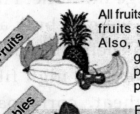

Don'ts
Foods to be avoided as far as possible

Flour Bags, rice, bread, refined flour, cornflower and its products, noodles, macaroni, spaghetti, chinese grass, etc.

Washed pulses or dals, green gram dal, red gram dal, bengal gram dal.

Do not remove edible skin and pips from fruits and eat in raw fresh stage rather than as cooked, tinned or juice.

Potato, sweet potato, over-cooked vegetables and cauliflower.

All condiments are permitted. Drink plenty of water during the day. Include one serving of fruit at each meal. Eat plenty of salad and vegetables at each meal.

Dietary fibre should not be increased suddenly as it may result in increased gas from the anus, belching, diarrhoea and feeling of fullness in the abdomen. *It is important to drink large quantities of fluid along with a high-fibre diet.* Constipation will worsen if you do not drink at least eight to ten glasses of water every day. If you have diseases of the kidney or heart, consult your doctor for the amount of water and other fluids you can drink per day.

- *Regular habits.* The best time for passing the stool is as soon as you get up in the morning or after a meal. Set aside at least ten to fifteen minutes every day, preferably in the morning, for passing the stool. You should do this even if there is no urge to pass stool. If you cannot pass it in the morning, try to set aside some time again during the day.

- *Posture*: The squatting posture (as with the Indian style toilet) with a narrow angle between the thighs and hips is the best posture for passing stool. This angle is absent in the western style toilet if either your feet hang above the floor, or if

Fig 2. Correct posture for passing the stool

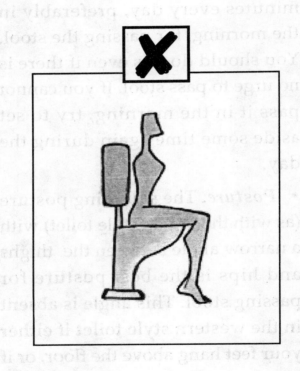

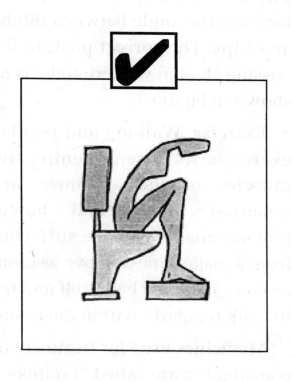

you are sitting straight. You can put a stool below the feet to increase the angle between thighs and hips. The correct posture for passing stool in western toilet is as shown in Figure 2.

- *Exercise*. Walking and regular exercises for strengthening the muscles of the abdomen are essential for normal bowel movements. If you are suffering from a major illness, move as often as you can on the bed itself and try to walk regularly within the room.

Medicines used for treatment of constipation are called *"laxatives"*.

Laxatives are medicines that increase peristalsis or alter consistency of the stool to facilitate its evacuation. Some laxatives which are inserted as capsules into the anus are called *"suppositories"*. Your doctor will prescribe medicines only if the symptoms are either severe or persist after regular practice of non-medicinal measures. Do not take laxatives without consulting your doctor. The duration of treatment will depend upon the severity of symptoms, associated diseases and dietary habits. Described below are the common groups of laxatives.

- ***Bulk agents.*** These are fibre supplements. Bulk agents are natural substances consisting of complex starch and cellulose. Commercially available fibre supplements are isafgula, methylcellulose, psyllium, and polycarbophil. Bulk agents normally have effect after about twelve to twenty-four hours and may take even a few days. *It is important to drink large quantities of water along with bulk agents.* Psyllium in the bulk agents

Fig 3. Mechanism of action of bulk laxatives

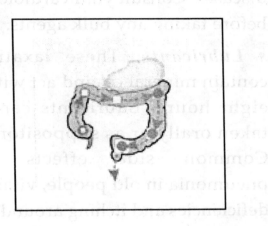

Bulk Laxatives

Absorb water, soften stools, increase stool volume and therefore increase peristalsis.

reduces the effect of some medicines recommended for heart diseases. Consult your cardiologist before taking any bulk agents.

• *Lubricants*. These laxatives contain mineral oil and act within eight hours. Lubricants can be taken orally or as suppositories. Common side effects are pneumonia in old people, vitamin deficiencies and itching around the anus. Lubricants are not recommended for pregnant women. They are not used regularly for treatment of constipation.

Fig 4. Mechanism of action of lubricants

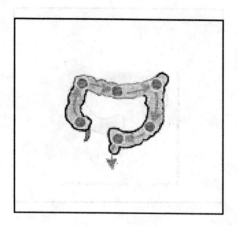

Lubricants
Help the stools to move smoothly in the intestine. They can also decrease water absorption.

Fig 5. Mechanism of action of stool softners

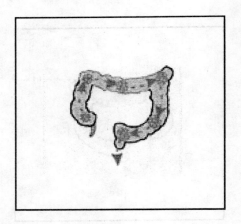

Stool Softners
Add moisture to the stools and make them soft. They may also increase water in the large intestine.

- *Stool softeners*. These laxatives contain docusate. They act within three days. Stool softeners are not habit forming and have very few side effects. They can interact with mineral oils and increase their absorption. They are therefore not recommended along with lubricant laxatives.

- *Saline laxatives*. Commonly used saline laxatives are magnesium citrate, sulphate and hydroxide, lactulose, sodium phosphate and glycerin suppositories. Saline laxatives are effective if immediate evacuation

Fig 6. Mechanism of action of saline laxatives

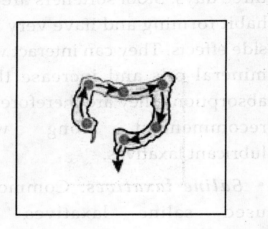

Saline Laxatives
Absorb water into the intestine, increase stool volume and therefore increase peristalsis.

of the bowel is required. They evacuate the stool within three hours if taken orally and within fifteen minutes if taken as suppositories.

Glycerin suppositories are often used before endoscopy procedure and for evacuation of hard stool from the rectum. These suppositories also lubricate the stool and stimulate the rectum to pass stool. Saline laxatives should not be taken regularly and avoided in people with kidney and heart diseases, high blood pressure, and distended large intestine.

- ***Stimulant laxatives.*** Bisacodyl, castor oil, senna and phenolphthalein are commonly used stimulant laxatives. They act within six to ten hours if taken orally and one hour if inserted as a suppository. Regular use of these laxatives results in dependency and loss of normal bowel function. They are not recommended in people with gall bladder diseases and ulcers in the large intestine. Stimulant laxatives are recommended in pregnancy. They reduce the effect of antacids. Common side effect is cramp-like pain in the abdomen.

Fig 7. Mechanism of action of stimulant laxatives

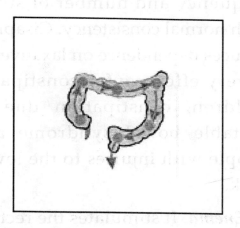

Stimulant Laxatives
Increase peristalsis. Some medicines in this group also increase water in the large intestine.

- ***Cisapride***. This medicine is not a laxative. It increases stool frequency and number of stools with normal consistency. Cisapride reduces dependence on laxatives. It is very effective for constipated children, constipation due to irritable bowel syndrome and people with injuries to the lower back.

- ***Enema***. It stimulates the rectum and thereby increases peristalsis in the large intestine. Enema is usually recommended if the stool is hard and lodged in the rectum. This is often observed in elderly people. Most of these people do not respond to laxatives. Enema is also used to evacuate the stool within a short time. Commonly used enema is soap water solution.

Hirschsprung's disease is treated with surgery. Benefits of the surgery are observed both in children and adults as normal functions of the rectum and anal sphincters.

Constipation in children. Children who suffer from regular constipation should be examined by a doctor to rule out any associated disease. If the child is normal, simple measures such as regular habits and dietary changes will prevent constipation. You should encourage children to develop healthy bowel habits very early in life. Instead of scolding them during toilet training, gently and firmly encourage them to try and pass the stool at a regular time every day. Similarly, instead of forcing the child to eat a high fibre diet, offer healthy food very frequently. Do not scold the child if you feel that he/she has not eaten "enough" nutritious food. Avoid keeping "junk" food in the house and within easy access of the children.

AYURVEDA

AYURVEDA

According to the Ayurveda, constipation is a disease where the stool is very hard with a predominance of "*vata*". According to the basic principles of Ayurveda, vata is one of the three *doshas* in the body. It is a combination of ether and air elements of the universe. Vata is responsible for movement and feeling in the whole body, including in the cells. This type of vata disorder is called ***anaha*** which means distention of the abdomen and its obstruction.

According to Ayurveda, constipation is the result of slow accumulation of *ama* or "immature" and undigested food and *purisa* which means the stool in the large intestine. This accumulation is due to aggravation of vata.

What are the symptoms of constipation?

There are two types of constipation:

- *amaja*, due to accumulation of immature and undigested food; and

- *purisaja*, due to accumulation of the stool and urine. Symptoms of *amaja* type of constipation are: thirst, uneasy feeling in the head, pain in the abdomen, suppression of belching and nausea. Symptoms of *purisaja* type of constipation are: pain in the abdomen, giddiness, vomiting of the undigested food, distention of the abdomen, bad smell and vomiting.

What are the causes of constipation?

Causes of constipation are broadly divided into five groups. These are:

- *Diet (Aharjanya).* Eating food which makes you feel very heavy and full, dry and rough food, and food which is very cold and kept after cooking for a long time are the common causes of constipation. In addition, eating food which is bitter and pungent also causes constipation.

- *Life-style (Viharajanya).* Suppression of natural urges, excessive physical exercise, inadequate sleep at night, consumption of alcohol and excess of sexual activity can also lead to constipation.

- *Environment (Asatmyajanya).* Eating food that does not agree with you, facing head winds, smoking and exposure to heat cause constipation.

- *Psychological (Manasajanya).* Mental diseases, grief, sorrow and fear result in constipation.

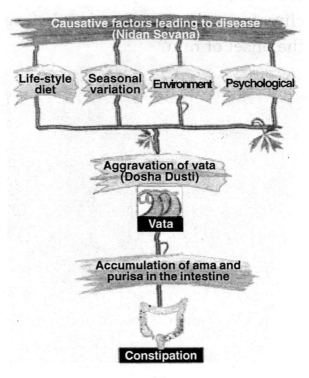

Fig 8. Ayurvedic philosophy of mechanism of development of constipation

- ***Season (Ritujanya).*** Some people get constipation whenever there is abnormality in the normal climate for the season or just before the onset of rain.

What is the treatment of constipation?

People with purisaja type of constipation (when stool accumulates in the intestine and blocks it) need to be hospitalized. Constipation of amaja type (due to undigested food) can be treated either with *single medicine* or with *group of medicines*. The duration of treatment and choice of medicine will depend upon the duration and cause of constipation. Your doctor is the best person to chose the type of medication required for your constipation.

Single medicines are:

- *Fruit pulp of cassia*. Taking this medicine with water twice a day gives relief from simple constipation. It is a mild laxative and also has a "cooling" effect. This medicine softens the stool and increases peristalsis.

- *Fruit rind of small chebulic myrobalan*. This medicine has to be taken with rock salt at bed time. Chebulic myrobalan is a mild laxative. It increases peristalsis.

Compound medicines or group of medicines commonly used for treatment of constipation are:

- *Triphala churna*. This medicine is very effective for people suffering from chronic constipation. It contains extracts from three plants: chebulic, belleric and embelic myrobalan. Of these, chebulic myrobalan is the laxative. The other two medicines reduce the adverse impact of chebulic myrobalan such as are increased gas and cramp-like pain in the abdomen. This medicine is usually taken with warm water twice a day.

- *Rasonadi vati*. One or two tablets of rasonadi vati taken with warm water twice a day is effective for curing chronic constipation.
- *Haritakikhanda*. This medicine should also be taken twice a day with warm water.
- *Sukumara ghritta*. This medicine is prepared in ghee and should be taken with a glass of milk twice a day.

Local applications recommended for treatment of constipation are:

- *Asafoetida*. Application of asafoetida or hing paste around the umbilicus gives relief from simple constipation of recent origin.

• *Mixed application*. A paste prepared from equal parts of saltpetre or nitrate of potash, fruit rind of embelic myrobalan, amonium chloride and black sesame applied around the umbilicus results in passing the stool. It also reduces gas in the intestine.

What is the recommended diet for constipation?

Wheat or rice with bran, vegetables and fruits, especially citrus fruits are recommended for management of constipation. Foods particularly recommended are: old rice (*Puranasali*), green gram, garlic, banana, bathua leaves, parmal (a vegetable), lemon, yam, and papaya.

What are the aggravating factors?

Ayurveda prohibits some foods and life-style for people suffering from constipation. Bitter, spicy, sour, dry and rough food aggravate constipation. You should therefore avoid their consumption. Other foods which should not be consumed include pulses, diets rich in fat and any other food that normally makes you feel unwell. Facing head-winds, suppression of natural urges, especially the urge to pass the stool, lack of sleep in the night and excess of sex worsen constipation.

HOMOEOPATHY

HOMEOPATHY

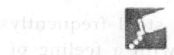

Criteria for defining constipation and its causes as per Homoeopathic system of medicine are the same as those described in the section on Allopathy. People who have constipation have one or more of the following symptoms:

• Incomplete passing of the stool;

• A feeling of inadequate passing of the stool. This feeling can be present even if there is no residual stool in the intestine or there is no urge to pass more stool;

- Passing the stool frequently accompanied with a feeling of fullness in the abdomen;
- Excessive straining to pass soft stool;
- Small volume of the stool (as compared to normal volume of the person) accompanied with gas.

Regular use of laxatives is discouraged in Homoeopathy. This is because of the possibility of laxative dependence. This dependence can be avoided by giving up laxatives for a few days periodically or changing the type of laxative. It is important to remember that you should not take any laxative without consulting your doctor.

What are the consequences of constipation?

Homoeopathy, just as in Ayurveda and Nature Cure, considers constipation as the root cause of several other illnesses. Common consequences of long-standing constipation are:

• Low resistance to various diseases;

• Early development of diseases which are at an early stage where symptoms have not yet started;

- Discomfort in the abdomen due to "gas";
- Allergies;
- Migraine; and
- Infections and other diseases of the digestive system.

What is the treatment of constipation?

A high-fibre diet is the most important measure for preventing and controlling constipation. Specific dietary recommendations are:

• *Drinking water*. You should drink about seven to eight glasses of water per day. Do not drink cold water with meals because it reduces temperature in the abdomen. Reduced temperature results in indigestion and therefore constipation.

- *Vegetables and fruits*. You should eat at least one bowl full of salads and fruits every day.

- *Avoid non-vegetarian food*. Non-vegetarian food is low in fibre and rich in fat. Regular intake of non-vegetarian food causes constipation.

- *Warm fluids*. Drinking hot milk, honey or lemon in hot water as soon as you get up in the morning stimulates peristalsis. A morning walk after taking these warm fluids enhances their effect.

- ***Stop smoking.*** Smoking or drinking tea or coffee result in constipation.

- ***Enema*** is recommended for people with severe constipation and in those who need quick relief from the discomfort of constipation. Enema should not be taken without doctor's advice.

What are the recommended Homoeopathic medicines for constipation?

There are no laxatives for treatment of constipation in the Homeopathic system. This is because the medicines are prescribed for the totality of symptoms including mental and personal life situations. For example a child may constipation due to fissure in the anus. This fissure may be the result of passing constipated hard stools. In such cases treatment of the fissure completely cures constipation.

Medicines for constipation in Homoeopathy are numerous. This is because the medicines are prescribed for the totality of symptoms. Your doctor will prescribe medicines, if necessary, only after taking detailed history. Some common medicines recommended for simple constipation without any associated diseases are:

- ***Nux vomica 6***. You should take this medicine at bed time. Nux vomica 6 is recommended for constipation of recent origin and after a heavy meal which is likely to result in discomfort and constipation. It is a very safe medicine.

- ***Mother biochemic combination No. 4***. This medicine is also effective for constipation of recent origin.

- ***Baryta carb 30***. This medicine is very effective for old people who have poor peristalsis and muscle tome.

- *Alumina 30*. This medicine is very effective for people who eat food cooked in aluminium vessels. This type of food results in decreased peristalsis.

It is important to remember that you should consult your doctor immediately if you have (1) pain or distention of the abdomen, (2) nausea and constipation at the same time.

How long should the medicines be taken?

The duration of treatment with Homoeopathic medicines depends upon the duration of constipation and other associated diseases. Simple constipation of recent origin can be cured with Homoeopathic medicines within ten to fifteen days. Treatment for three months to one year may be necessary for chronic and/or severe constipation even if it is not associated with other diseases. Regular intake of high-fibre diet reduces the duration of treatment.

NATURE CURE

NATURE CURE

Nature Cure philosophy considers constipation as one of the important causes of several diseases such as appendicitis, rheumatism, arthritis, high blood pressure and cancer. This is because of the theory that "poisons" are formed from stools if they are not passed out regularly. This "poison" enters the blood and weakens the vital organs of the body. It also lowers the resistance to various diseases.

Constipation results in other associated problems such as

- accumulation of "gas" in the abdomen,
- a feeling of fullness in the stomach,
- lack of appetite,
- irritability,
- anxiety and
- lack of concentration.

All the fruits and vegetables peels!! She must love the cow more than her family

What is constipation?

Constipation is defined in Nature Cure as inadequate movement of bowels or inability of the intestine to pass the stool. According to this system of medicine you do not have constipation if:

• you are able to pass the stool as soon as you get up in the morning;

• the entire process of passing the stool does not take more than a few moments;

• the stool is straw in colour, long like a thread, cylindrical in shape and without smell;

- the stool does not dirty the area around the anus;

- you feel light in the stomach after passing the stool; and

- you pass the stool with the above characteristics twice a day.

Very few people fulfil the above criteria. According to Nature Cure principles, you have partial constipation if you fulfil at least two of the above criteria. Causes of constipation described in Nature Cure are the same as those detailed in the section on Allopathy.

What is the treatment of constipation?

It is important to identify the cause of constipation and treat it for complete cure of constipation. Detailed below is management of simple constipation without any associated diseases.

Drinking water. You should drink at least ten to twelve glasses of water every day. Water provides relief because:

- it maintains the moisture in the intestine and makes the stool soft;

- water absorbs the "heat" generated from long-standing stool in the abdomen; and

- water increases volume of the stool.

Drinking four to five glasses of water as soon as you get up in the morning also relieves constipation. It is important to remember that you should not drink water with meals as it dilutes stomach juices essential for digestion. Dilution of stomach juices causes indigestion and therefore constipation. You should drink water half an hour before and after meals.

Mud pack. A smooth paste of pure clay obtained about ten centimetres below the surface of the earth is prepared in warm water. This paste is applied on a strip of cloth. The usual size of the abdominal mud pack is twenty centimetres long, ten centimetres wide and two and a half centimetres thick. Keep the mud pack on the abdomen and cover it with a blanket. This pack is usually applied for ten to thirty minutes. Mud pack reduces "heat" from the abdomen and breaks morbid matter in the abdomen.

Cold towel pack. A towel dipped in cold water can be kept on the abdomen for about ten to thirty minutes instead of a mud pack.

Cold hip bath. This bath includes keeping the waist region in a special tub partially filled with cold water for fifteen minutes. After the bath lie down in a bed covered with blankets. Cold hip bath removes "poisons" from the stomach.

Massage. An abdominal massage is very useful for relief from constipation. It stimulates peristalsis, tones muscles of the abdomen and evacuates the stool. You should do the abdominal massage about two hours after meals. It is important for you to learn the correct method of massage from a Nature Cure practitioner.

Abdominal massage should not be given to people having any type of hernia, inflammation of the female reproductive organs, stones in the kidneys, bladder or gall bladder, ulcers, high blood pressure and during pregnancy.

Abdominal pack. Keeping a cloth dipped in cold water on the abdomen for twenty minutes increases blood circulation in the abdomen. Increased blood circulation improves digestion and forms normal consistency of the stool. This pack should be used three hours after dinner every day.

Enema. A warm water enema gives quick relief from constipation, especially if the hard stool is located in the lower part of the large intestine. Sometimes an oil is injected into the rectum before going to bed. This oil lubricates the rectum and makes the stool pass out smoothly. You should not take enema unless the doctor recommends it.

Douche. Washing the anal region with cold water stimulates peristalsis.

Regular habit. You should devote some time for passing the stool every morning as soon as you get up. This should be done even if you do not have an urge to pass the stool.

What is the recommended diet for constipation?

You should eat a regular high fibre diet with less fat and moderate protein. An ideal diet is one which has seventy percent green leafy and other vegetable, salads and soups and thirty percent cereals. Citrus fruits have natural laxatives and therefore should be eaten every day.

A high fibre diet alone is not enough to prevent constipation. It is important that you chew every mouthful of food at least fifteen times. You should also avoid irregular meals. Isabgol, a bulk agent is a safe and effective laxative. Specific dietary recommendations for relief from constipation are:

Fruits. Most fruits except banana and jack fruit relieve constipation. Bael fruit is considered to be the best laxative. It has dual properties. It makes hard stool soft and loose stools such as in diarrhoea hard. Eating about sixty grams of the fruit before dinner for two to three months gives complete relief from constipation. Pear, prunes, grapes and guava are also effective laxatives. They should be eaten either after dinner or with breakfast

Prunes are rich in soluble fibre. However, their laxative effect is not dependant on the fibre alone. Prune juice is also a very effective laxative. Prunes can result in gas and abdominal disturbances if you start eating them in large quantities suddenly. Start eating one small portion of the fruit initially and gradually increase the quantity till your bowel movements are normal.

Grapes improve the muscle tone of the stomach and intestines. About three hundred and fifty grams of grapes should be eaten everyday. If fresh grapes are not available, raisins soaked in water for twenty four hours should be eaten along with the soaked water every morning.

Vegetables. Peas, potato, sweet potato, beet root, all green leafy vegetables, beans, carrots, cabbage, bottle gourd, tinda, and snake gourd are recommended for people suffering from constipation.

Wheat bran. About three tablespoons of wheat bran from the mill is adequate to maintain normal bowel movements. You can add this bran to the wheat flour while making rotis. Wheat bran is one of the most effective and easily available natural laxative which increases the bulk of the stool and keeps it soft.

You should avoid food such as refined wheat flour (maida), fried food and fast food. You should also avoid drinking tea or coffee.

Exercise. A combination of regular high-fibre diet and exercise is essential for normal bowel movements. Exercise improves peristalsis and tones abdominal muscles. Walking at least three to four kilometres a day improves bowel movements.

Regular practice of yoga also relieves constipation. Yoga increases peristalsis and strengthens abdominal and pelvic muscles. Yoga and meditation are particularly effective for people suffering from Irritable Bowel Syndrome.

HEALTH TIP

High fibre diet has several advantages. In addition to preventing constipation, it reduces cholesterol and the likelihood of development of some cancers, especially cancer of the intestine. It is, therefore recommended that you eat a high-fiber diet even if you do not have constipation.

Definitions

Anus is the outer opening of the digestive canal through which the stool is passed out of the body.

Biopsy is removal of a small part of living tissue from an organ for examination under a microscope. It is used to establish diagnosis and estimate progress of the disease or treatment.

Diaphragm is a dome-shaped muscular partition that separates the chest and abdomen. It moves up and down during breathing.

Enzyme is a protein produced by living cells. Digestive enzymes are produced in large quantities and act in the digestive canal.

Hereditary diseases are diseases that are transmitted from parents to the children.

Intestine is a coiled tubular tube which extends from the stomach to the anus. It is divided into small and large intestine.

Laxatives are medicines which increase bowel movements, soften the stool and cause evacuation of the stool.

Peristalsis is a coordinated, rhythmic, and serial contraction of the intestine that pushes food forward.

Rectum is the last part of the large intestine.

Suppositories are medicines that cause evacuation of the stool and are inserted into the rectum.

References

Allopathy

Kreek M J and J A Culpepper-Morgan, Constipation syndromes: In: A pharmacologic approach to gastrointestinal disorders. Ed JH Lewis 1994. Pp 179-208.

Martelli H. Devroede G, Arhan P et al (1978). Some parameters of large bowel motility in normal man. Gastroenterology, 75, 612-18.

Reynolds J C, Ouyang A, Lee C A

et al (1987) Chronic severe constipation: Prospective motility studies in 25 consecutive patients. Gastroenterology, 92, 414-20.

Sleisenger and Fortran; Gastrointestinal diseases: Pathophysiology, diagnosis and management, Vol. I. Pp 837-887.

Ayurveda

A hand book of domestic medicines and common Ayurvedic remedies, Published by Central Council for Research in Ayurveda and Siddha, New Delhi.

Bhaisajya Ratnavali
Charaka Samhita
Madhava Chikitsa
Madhava Nidana
Susruta Samhita